WHAT EVERY PROVIDER SHOULD KNOW

A Trauma-Informed Guide for Healthcare Professionals

Marie McKenzie

MARIE L MCKENZIE LLC

ISBN: 979-8-9884482-7-3 – Paperback

ISBN: 979-8-9884482-9-7 – Hard Cover

ISBN: 979-8-9884482-8-0 - eBook

For permissions, workshops, or bulk purchases, please contact: Marie L McKenzie LLC at marielmckenzie@gmail.com

Disclaimer:
The information provided in this book is intended for educational and informational purposes only. It is not a substitute for medical, legal, or mental health advice, diagnosis, or treatment. Healthcare providers are encouraged to follow institutional protocols, professional guidelines, and applicable laws and regulations when implementing trauma-informed practices.

While every effort has been made to ensure the accuracy and relevance of the content, the author and publisher make no guarantees regarding outcomes or results from the use of this material.

The experiences, scenarios, and stories shared throughout this book are based on real clinical insights and survivor narratives. Some examples have been modified or fictionalized to protect privacy and confidentiality.

The views expressed in this book are those of the author and do not reflect the policies or positions of any affiliated organizations or institutions.

Reader discretion is advised, especially for those who may find discussions of trauma or sexual violence triggering.

Contents

Dedication

Every survivor who has ever stayed silent, unsure if they would be believed,

To the providers who choose compassion over convenience, presence over protocol; thank you for being the difference.

And to the younger me, who once needed the care I now teach others to give;You didn't give up.You rose.

Foreword

"Leadership isn't about being in charge; it is about creating an environment to inspire others to be their very best, especially in times when it is most needed, when compassionate ideas feel safe to grow".

Nowhere is this truth more vital than in the work of caring for trauma survivors. In spaces where pain, loss, and vulnerability are ever-present, leadership must become less about authority and more about stewardship by cultivating trust, safety, and hope in the soil of human experience.

True leadership in trauma is the courage to listen before speaking, to hold silence without rushing to fill it, and to see the person behind the pain. It is a form of leadership that values connection over control, empathy over efficiency, and healing over hierarchy. It is about recognizing that every survivor and every member of the healthcare team carries a story and that those stories shape the way we see, serve, and show up in the world. In truth, every person in healthcare is a leader, a leader for the patients we are privileged to serve.

Compassionate leadership calls us to build environments where people feel safe to bring their full selves, where their voices matter, their experiences are honored, and their potential is nurtured. It's about leading not from above, but alongside; not by command, but through care. As HCA Healthcare founding father, Tommy Frist Sr., wisely said, *"Good people beget good people".*

This book offers a vision of leadership that is profoundly human. It challenges the traditional models that equate power with dominance and replaces them with frameworks rooted in understanding, relational safety, and shared purpose. It reminds us that trauma informed care isn't only a clinical approach, it's a way of leading, living, and belonging.

As you turn these pages, may you find both inspiration and invitation: to lead with heart, to listen with humility, and to create spaces where healing and innovation grow side by side. For in the end, leadership is not about titles or tasks, it is about tending the ground where others can thrive, where compassion becomes culture, and where every act of care becomes a seed of change.

In compassion and purpose,

John Gerhold, MSHCM, R.T.(R)

CEO - HCA Florida Lake Monroe Hospital

Acknowledgements

I extend my deepest gratitude to the survivors whose strength and courage continue to inspire my work. Your stories are the heartbeat of this book, and the reason trauma-informed care must remain at the center of every healthcare interaction. And to the healthcare professionals who continue to show up with compassion and courage every day, I see you.

To My George, whose unwavering love, patience, and encouragement make it possible for me to keep showing up for this mission.

To my family and friends, thank you for your love, encouragement, and belief in my work. Your prayers, kind words, and steady support carried me through the long hours of writing and reflection. Each of you has played a special part in this journey, reminding me that purpose is nurtured through community and love. I'm forever grateful for your presence in my life.

My heartfelt appreciation goes to my colleagues at the Florida Council Against Sexual Violence (FCASV) and the Victim Service Center of Central Florida (VSC) for their continued leadership, advocacy, and dedication to trauma-informed care.

To J.L. Campbell, my editor, thank you for your keen insight and dedication to excellence.

I'm deeply grateful to my incredible team of beta readers for their time, insight, encouragement, and belief in this mission. Your thoughtful feedback made this work stronger and more impactful.

And finally, to every healthcare professional who chooses compassion over convenience and presence over protocol, thank you for being part of the change.

Introduction

Why This Book, Why Now?

I've been a nurse for more than twenty-six years. I've cared for trauma survivors in the chaos of emergency rooms, in the quiet of exam rooms in the community setting, and in the stillness that follows a disclosure. I've also lived through trauma myself; long before I wore scrubs or learned what it meant to be trauma-informed.

That's why this work isn't just professional. It's personal.

Over the years, I've seen a dangerous gap in healthcare:

We are trained to save lives, but not always to hold stories.

We know how to stop bleeding, start IVs, perform procedures, and prescribe medication.

But few of us are ever taught how to recognize trauma, or how to respond with compassion when it's silently standing in the waiting room, sitting on the exam table, hospital bed, or ER stretcher.

Sexual violence is more common than most people realize. Survivors come into our clinics, hospitals, dental offices, school health rooms, and private practices every single day. They're not always ready to say what happened. But they're watching to see how we treat them. They are listening for safety in our tone. Measuring trust in our eyes. Searching for proof they won't be dismissed or hurt again.

Too often, they leave re-traumatized.

Not because we don't care; but because we weren't given the tools.

That's what this book is here to do—change the narrative.

Who This Book Is For

This book is for all healthcare providers and teams, not just trauma specialists.

It's for:

- The dental hygienist who notices a patient flinch at "open wide"
- The pediatrician who doesn't know why a child won't speak
- The OBGYN who senses fear behind a forced smile
- The ER nurse who feels helpless when a patient cries during triage
- The front desk staff who doesn't understand why someone storms out
- The medical director trying to lead a team through burnout and fear

Whether you're a physician, nurse, medical assistant, therapist, administrator, security personnel, transporter, or technician—any member of the healthcare team—you are a potential safe space for a survivor. And whether you realize it or not, many of them are already walking through your doors.

What This Book Offers

Inside, you'll find a trauma-informed care framework I call R.I.S.E. Designed to help providers care for every patient with dignity and safety, regardless of whether a disclosure is made. It stands for:

- R – Recognize the Signs of Trauma
- I – Initiate Safety Care
- S – Support Healing
- E – Empower Recovery

In the chapters ahead we'll walk through each of these pillars in detail—with practical tools, real-life scenarios, specialty-specific examples, and language you can use immediately. You'll also find scripts, checklists, prayers, and protocols to guide you, your team, and your organization toward becoming more survivor-centered in every encounter. And because caring for survivors also requires caring for ourselves, chapter nine focuses on provider self-care—helping you build resilience, set healthy boundaries, and sustain compassion in this important work.

A Note to the Reader

This is not a book that shames. It is a book that equips. You don't need to be perfect. You don't need to have a background in trauma therapy. You just need to be willing to show up with presence, humility, and care.

If you've ever felt unsure what to say when someone discloses...

If you've ever wondered why certain patients act in confusing or difficult ways...

If you've ever wanted to care better, but didn't know how...

This book is for you.

Together, we can create safer spaces. Together, we can change the experience of healthcare; for survivors and for ourselves.

Together, we can rise.

Chapter One

Understanding Trauma And The Survivor Experience

Trauma doesn't always scream. Sometimes it whispers through clenched jaws, flinching shoulders, and a gaze that won't meet yours. It enters the exam room long before the provider—and lingers long after the appointment ends.

As a nurse, I've seen it in the quiet teen who nods without speaking. I've heard it in the story that unravels during a routine visit, when the weight of silence becomes too heavy for the patient to carry alone. And as a survivor, I know what it means to sit on an exam table, unsure if my body is safe in someone else's hands.

That's why trauma-informed care isn't optional. It's essential.

Trauma Is Not Just What Happened. It's How It Landed

Trauma isn't defined solely by events; it's defined by *impact*. Two people can experience the same situation and carry completely different burdens. What makes something traumatic isn't just its severity; it's the sense of powerlessness, isolation, and the threat it creates inside the nervous system.

For sexual assault survivors, trauma is not just in the memory. It's in the body—in hypervigilance, in flinching at touch, in not being able to sit still during a pelvic exam, or freezing when asked to remove a gown.

All patients, regardless of age, gender, or reason for visit, must be approached with the understanding that trauma may be part of their story. Because statistically, it likely is.

What Every Provider Should Know

- Nearly 1 in 3 women and about 1 in 4 men experience sexual violence in their lifetime.
- Every 74 seconds someone in the USA is sexually assaulted. Every nine minutes, that someone is a child.
- Sexual abuse affects all races, ages, religions, and socioeconomic backgrounds.
- Most survivors never disclose. Those who do often share for the first time in healthcare settings.
- Common survivor responses include dissociation, flat affect, anxiety, resistance, people-pleasing, or shutdown.
- Early trauma, including Adverse Childhood Experiences (ACEs), can shape how individuals respond to stress, relationships, and medical environments across the lifespan.

And yet, most healthcare providers receive little to no training on how to recognize or respond to specific situations.

To close this gap, trauma-informed care provides a universal framework that helps every provider understand not just what trauma looks like, but how to respond safely and effectively.

The 4R's of Trauma-Informed Care (SAMHSA, 2014)

These foundational principles, adapted from the Substance Abuse and Mental Health Services Administration (SAMHSA) model, provide a lens through which all care should be delivered:

1. **Realize** the widespread nature of trauma.

2. **Recognize** the signs in patients, families, and staff.

3. **Respond** by applying trauma knowledge in policies and practices.

4. **Resist Re-Traumatization** by eliminating harmful routines or language.

Throughout this book, these "4 Rs" will serve as a compass. But to make them practical and specialty-specific, we'll anchor them in a framework I teach in my training: **R.I.S.E.**

Introducing the R.I.S.E. Framework

R.I.S.E. was developed to fill a critical gap in how we teach trauma-informed care to healthcare teams. While many frameworks offer good theory, R.I.S.E. goes further—offering practical, heart-centered tools that providers can begin applying from day one.

Each pillar is simple but powerful:

- **R – Recognize the Signs of Trauma**
- **I – Initiate Safety Care**
- **S – Support Healing**
- **E – Empower Recovery**

You'll see this framework woven throughout the book—not only in direct patient care but in communication, documentation, follow-up, and team protocols.

A Story That Stays With Me

A young woman came to the ER one night for abdominal pain. She was quiet, withdrawn, and wouldn't let us examine her thoroughly. Another nurse rolled her eyes when the patient refused the pelvic exam. "She's wasting our time," the nurse muttered.

But I saw the fear in the woman's eyes. I sat beside her and gently asked, "Has anything ever happened to you that would make this kind of exam feel scary?" She burst into tears. She had been assaulted at 14 and hadn't told anyone—not even her family.

In that moment, I wasn't just her nurse. I was the first person she trusted with her truth.

That night helped to change how I practiced. I stopped assuming silence meant consent. I stopped seeing resistance as rudeness. And I began encouraging others to do the same.

Why This Matters in Every Specialty

You may not be a member of the ER team. You might be a pediatrician, dentist, OBGYN, school nurse, or chiropractor. You might be a family doctor with 20 patients to see before lunch. But no matter what your title or your practice setting, this truth holds:

You may be the only safe person a survivor sees this year. Maybe in their lifetime.

Will your care invite trust? Or unknowingly re-open a wound?

Reflection: What Do You Bring Into the Room?

Take a moment to consider:

- What assumptions do I carry about patients who seem "difficult"?
- Have I ever dismissed or misunderstood trauma responses as behavioral issues?
- How do I respond when I feel rushed, triggered, or uncomfortable?

Awareness is the first step toward being trauma-informed.

A Provider's Prayer

God, let my presence be soft,
my hands be gentle,
my tone be steady.
Let me see beyond symptoms.
Let me hold sacred what they don't say.
Amen.

Chapter Two

Recognize the Signs of Trauma (R)

A compassionate lens for every provider in every setting

Trauma rarely walks in holding a sign. It doesn't always come with a clear history or a diagnosis code. It shows up in the things we're trained to overlook—missed appointments, vague complaints, resistance, silence.

We're taught to treat what's visible. But trauma demands we listen to what's not being said.

"Recognize" is the first pillar of the R.I.S.E. framework because it changes how we *see*.

When you begin to recognize the signs of trauma, you shift from reacting to patient behavior to responding to their experience.

This is where trauma-informed care begins.

Trauma in Disguise

Trauma doesn't always look like crisis. In fact, many survivors become masters of survival, appearing compliant, cheerful, or even overly grateful. Others may seem oppositional, distracted, avoidant, or anxious.

Without trauma-informed training, these behaviors are easy to misinterpret.

Common signs that may indicate trauma:

- Flinching at touch or sudden movements

- Flat affect, dissociation, or zoning out during exams
- Disproportionate fear or panic in response to routine procedures
- Difficulty with authority, eye contact, or personal space
- Aggression, withdrawal, excessive people-pleasing
- Somatic complaints with no clear cause (chronic pain, GI issues)
- A history of frequent doctor/hospital visits or changing providers
- Overexplaining or apologizing excessively

Trauma isn't always "emotional." It's physiological. It lives in the body, and the body remembers.

Across the Spectrum: What It Might Look Like

Let's explore what trauma might look like in different specialties and settings:

Pediatrics & Adolescent Care

In the bright light of a pediatrician's office, a ten-year-old child avoids all eye contact and won't speak during a routine visit. Her guardian explains she's "just shy." She flinches when asked to remove her shirt for the exam and becomes unusually still when the provider touches her arm. This isn't just shyness; it's survival mode.

Red flags: sudden stillness, extreme avoidance, discomfort with bodily exposure, dissociation during exam.

Some kids don't have the language for what happened to them. Silence is how they survive.

Dentistry & Oral Surgery

She sat in the dental chair, hands gripping the armrests so tightly her knuckles turned white. The dentist leaned in and said, *"Open wide."* She froze. Her mind wasn't in the room anymore, it was back in a dark bedroom, hearing those same words from the person who had abused her as a child. She didn't speak up. She endured the exam, holding her breath, counting the seconds until it was over. The provider didn't pause, didn't ask or offer reassurance. He never knew why she avoided making another appointment.

Moments like this are why trauma-informed care is not optional. Even routine, everyday phrases can carry unexpected weight for someone with a history of sexual violence

Note: Language like "open wide," "it won't hurt," or "you're safe" can echo perpetrator phrases.

OBGYN & Reproductive Health

A patient refuses a pelvic exam, avoids scheduling pap smears, and tenses her entire body during breast exams. She appears agitated and defensive, even when spoken to gently.

Red flags: refusal of essential care, tension, avoidance of reproductive-related visits.

Primary Care/Internal Medicine

A 35-year-old woman attends her annual exam. She appears tense and avoids eye contact. During a routine question about her sexual history, she becomes tearful and changes the subject. The provider acknowledges her distress, offers to pause, and assures her that she is in control of the conversation. The patient later discloses a history of sexual assault and expresses relief at not being pressured.

Remember! Survivors may never disclose their history. Trauma-informed care ensures your practice is safe for both those who speak up and those who stay silent.

Scenario: Kayla, a Seventeen-Year-Old New Patient

Kayla arrives with her grandmother for a sports physical. She's quiet and cooperative—almost too cooperative. When the provider asks if she'd like her grandmother to step out, she quickly says "No, she can stay," then stares at the floor. During the abdominal exam, she stiffens and winces, even though the pressure is minimal.

When asked, "Is there anything else you'd like to talk about today?" Kayla shrugs and says, "Nope."

Later, the provider writes, "Patient denies concerns. Exam unremarkable." But trauma was in the room—and missed.

The Power of Noticing

Recognizing trauma doesn't require special tools. It requires presence, humility, and a shift in mindset:

From "What's wrong with you?" to "What happened to you? "From "They're noncompliant" to "They're protecting themselves."

This shift transforms frustration into compassion and confusion into clarity.

Affirmation for Providers: "Every behavior has a backstory. I choose to look deeper."

The Six Principles of Trauma-Informed Care (SAMHSA, 2014)

Recognizing trauma is just the beginning. To build truly trauma-informed environments, healthcare professionals must ground their care in the six core principles developed by the **Substance Abuse and Mental Health Services Administration (SAMHSA)**. In addition to the 4 Rs mentioned in Chapter One, these doctrines provide a framework for healing-centered systems of care—those that restore trust, safety, and connection.

1. **Safety**: Every patient and provider should feel physically and emotionally safe.

2. Trustworthiness and Transparency: Trust is earned through honesty, consistency, and open communication.

3. Peer Support: Healing is strengthened through connection and survivor-informed collaboration.

4. Collaboration and Mutuality — Healing happens in partnership; every voice has value.

5. Empowerment, Voice, and Choice: Survivors regain power through shared decision-making and validation.

6. Cultural, Historical, and Gender Awareness: Respecting identity, history, and cultural background is central to equitable, compassionate care.

Together, these six principles form the foundation of trauma-informed practice. They help providers shift from *"What's wrong with you?"* to *"What happened to you?"*—and ultimately to *"How can I help you feel safe right now?"*

Action Steps: What You Can Do Today

Practice Observational Awareness

Notice tone, posture, affect, body language, and interaction style. Take note of sudden changes in mood or physical response.

Avoid Assumptions

Don't assume compliance means comfort or that silence means consent. Survivors often mask discomfort to "get through it."

Create Space for Safety

Give patients permission to speak; or not. Use phrases like:

□ "You don't have to answer anything you're not comfortable with."

□ "Let me know if you'd like to pause."

□ "Would you like someone else in the room?"

Share Observations Gently

Instead of, "What's wrong?" try:

□ "I notice you seem uncomfortable; how can I help?"

□ "We can take this as slow as you need to."

Reflection:

- When a patient is "difficult," what assumptions do I make?
- Do I leave space for stories I may never hear?
- How often do I consider trauma as a possible factor in behavior?

Provider's Prayer

God, help me see with compassionate eyes.
Let me recognize what others have missed. T
each me to honor the silence as much as the story.
Let my presence say, "You are safe here."
Amen.

Chapter Three

Initiate Safe Care (I)

Every interaction is either an invitation or a warning.

When a survivor walks into a healthcare setting, they aren't just evaluating the provider. They're scanning the room for danger—consciously or unconsciously. They notice tone. Lighting. Positioning. Language. What's on the walls. Who's in the room. Who has power.

They are measuring *safety* with every breath. They are deciding if they feel safe enough to trust you.

For patients who've experienced sexual violence, the healthcare environment can feel like a replay of the trauma—disrobing, being touched, losing control, not understanding what's happening. Even when care is well-intentioned, it can still retraumatize if safety and trust aren't intentionally built into every interaction.

That's why the second pillar of R.I.S.E. is **Initiate Safe Care**, because survivors shouldn't have to earn safety. It's our job to offer it.

Safety Starts Before the Exam

Trauma-informed care doesn't begin when the provider walks in. It begins at the front desk. At check-in. In the waiting room. First contact is not just courtesy; it's a clinical intervention. A patient who feels safe is more likely to engage, comply with care plans, and participate in continued care beyond the visit.

Every staff member, from receptionist to security, medical assistant, scheduler, and nurse, can either build trust or unintentionally trigger fear.

What contributes to emotional or physical safety?

- A respectful tone and nonjudgmental eye contact
- Being asked before being touched, moved, or even addressed.
- An uncluttered, clean, warm environment
- A choice about who is in the room
- A door that closes fully or not, if needed
- A place to sit that feels safe and offers comfort
- A clearly stated plan for the visit: "Here's what you can expect today..."

Language That Builds and Breaks Trust

Words matter. Tone matters more.

Common phrases that may cause harm:

- "Relax, I've done this a thousand times."
- "It'll only take a second."
- "If you don't cooperate, we can't help you."
- "This won't hurt."
- "You're fine."

Even when spoken gently, these phrases remove autonomy and mimic language used by abusers.

Trauma-informed alternatives:

- "I'll walk you through everything before we begin."

- "Is it okay if we start now?"
- "You're in control. We can pause at any time."
- "Would you like me to explain each step as we go, or would you prefer quiet?"

Creating Safety in Your Physical Space

You don't need a major renovation to create a trauma-informed environment. Start small:

Clinic or Office Adjustments:

- Ensure gowns are adequate and offer coverage
- Allow patients to disrobe in private, not while someone waits in the room
- Keep doors fully closed or curtains drawn during exams
- Position yourself at eye level when speaking
- Avoid hovering, sudden movements, or standing over seated patients
- Use soft lighting when possible
- Display a visible, inclusive patient rights poster or "You're safe here" sign
- Offer a choice of music, silence, or distraction when appropriate

Patients don't just want safety. They want to feel safe.

Scenario: The Power of a Pause

Dr. Malik, a family medicine physician, enters the room of a 45-year-old woman scheduled for a breast exam. He smiles warmly, washes his hands, and says, "Let's get started." The patient stiffens but says nothing. When he reaches for her gown, she blurts out, "Can I have a female do this?"

He hesitates, then quietly replies, "Of course. Thank you for asking me." He steps out, asks a female nurse to take over, and returns later to check in.

Later in a follow-up note, the patient writes: *"I thought I'd have to endure it. I was surprised by how quickly they respected my request. That's never happened before."*

It's not always the grand gestures. It's the **gentle pivots** that build trust.

For Dental, Pediatric, and OB/GYN Providers

Every specialty has unique procedures, but the principles remain the same.

Dentistry

- Tell the patient **before** reclining the chair or placing instruments near the mouth.
- Avoid rushing intake and explain equipment and sounds before use.
- Ask, "Would you like me to explain everything, or just the basics?"
- Develop a plan for them to signal when they need a break (e.g., raising a hand).

Pediatrics

- Ask the child's permission before touching, when developmentally appropriate.
- Validate their discomfort: "It's okay to feel nervous. We're going to take our time."
- Avoid overpowering language like "Be a big girl/boy" or "You're being dramatic."

OBGYN

- Allow patients to insert the speculum themselves if desired; offer the option.

- Narrate each step and ask for permission before proceeding.
- Offer a support person, music, or grounding tools.

Action Steps for Creating Trust

Narrate the Visit: Patients should never be surprised by what's coming next.

Offer Options: "Would you prefer to sit or lie down?" "Would you like a nurse in the room?"

Validate, Don't Minimize: If someone appears anxious, say: "I can tell this feels difficult. Thank you for showing up today."

"Is there anything I can do to make you more comfortable?"

Respect Autonomy: If a patient refuses a procedure, **never pressure**. Provide more education about the procedure and ask how you can help. Ask what might help them feel more comfortable next time.

Reflection

- How do I normally begin my visits?
- Do I assume consent because the patient is present, or do I ask again?
- Do my body language and tone communicate respect?
- If I were the patient, would I feel in control?

Affirmation: "Every patient deserves to feel safe in my care." I offer trust before I expect it."

A Provider's Prayer

Lord, let me be a resting place.
Not just a provider, but a person who welcomes others with gentleness.
Remind me that kindness is clinical.
That consent is sacred.
That every interaction can be healing or harmful.
Help me choose healing.
Amen.

Chapter Four

Support Healing (S)

Because how we respond matters as much as what we do.

Most survivors don't expect a miracle in the exam room. They aren't asking you to erase what happened. But they are watching for one thing:

Will you believe me?

That's why the "S" in R.I.S.E. stands for **Support Healing**. Be nonjudgmental. It's not about fixing. It's about holding space without harm; offering neutrality, safety, and presence when someone risks revealing their pain.

Whether a disclosure is verbal, non-verbal, or never spoken at all, your response can shape whether a survivor feels safe enough to return or safe enough to reach out for support to heal.

What Support Looks Like in Practice

Support without judgment isn't complicated. But it does require intention.

It sounds like:

- "Thank you for trusting me with that."
- "I believe you."
- "That shouldn't have happened to you."
- "You're not alone."

- "Would you like to talk about options?"
- It **does not** sound like:
- "Are you sure?"
- "Why didn't you say something sooner?"
- "Do you want to report it?" (as the **first** response)
- "But you seem fine."
- "Let's not dwell on that. Let's get back to your exam."

Even subtle expressions such as raised eyebrows, awkward pauses, and silence can feel like disbelief to a survivor. Many have already endured blame, shame, or minimization. If your words echo those of past responders, it reinforces the message: "I shouldn't have said anything."

Disclosure Can Be Subtle

Most survivors won't say, "I was sexually assaulted." Instead, they may say:

- "I'm just nervous around men."
- "I don't like being touched."
- "I hate exams like this."
- "I've had a bad experience before."
- "I just want to get it over with."

These are invitations to respond with care, not interrogate or explain away their fears or issues.

Scenario: The Dental Chair Disclosure

Miguel, a 34-year-old man, comes in for a routine dental procedure. As the hygienist prepares the suction, he becomes visibly tense. When the dentist begins using the scaler,

Miguel grips the chair and says, "This reminds me of some stuff that happened years ago. Can we just wait a minute?"

Instead of brushing it off, the dentist pauses, lowers his tools, and says, "Absolutely. We can stop anytime you need. Thank you for letting me know." Miguel exhales. For the first time, he feels seen; not just treated.

This isn't about the perfect response. It's about showing up, offering calm support, empathy, and giving control back.

When Support Means Saying Less

One of the most trauma-informed things you can do is **not rush to fill the silence.** Survivors don't need you to solve the pain. They need you to hold it with them, if only for a moment.

"When I finally told someone, they didn't try to fix it. They just said, 'I'm so sorry that happened.' And that was enough."—Survivor

When You Feel Uncomfortable

Disclosures can stir discomfort, uncertainty, or even memories of your own unresolved history. That's normal.

Here's what you can do:

- Pause. Breathe. Stay grounded.
- Acknowledge without digging. You're not an investigator. You're a caregiver.
- Offer resources. You can say, "Would it be helpful if I gave you information about someone you can talk to?"

The Impact of Judgment-Free Support

Survivors often remember the first person who listened without disbelief. That moment can be a turning point; where shame loses power and healing begins.

You may never know what that interaction meant. But it matters more than you think.

Specialty Considerations

Internal Medicine/Primary Care

- Avoid assumptions based on presentation (e.g., "You don't *look* like a trauma survivor."
- Offer gentle options like, "We can stop, or do a different part of the exam first."

Pediatrics

- Let children lead. Ask before touching. Use developmentally appropriate words.
- Believe disclosures even when they seem fragmented. Children and even adults often share in pieces.

Dentistry

- Respond to verbal and body cues with compassion: "We don't have to do this today."
- Let patients choose their pace. Offer breaks often.

Mental Health Providers

- Trauma may surface mid-session, even if not part of the initial complaint.
- Reflect safety, not shock. "That took courage to share."

Action Steps

Normalize disclosures

Use language that invites honesty: "This is a safe space. You don't have to share more than you want to, but I'm here to listen if you do."

Respond neutrally and supportively

Whether you believe it "makes sense" or not, your job is not to evaluate; it's to validate.

Offer resources, not ultimatums

Say, "There are people who can support you if you'd like. Would you like their contact information?"

Practice reflective listening.

Mirror their emotion without taking over. "It sounds like that was really painful. I'm so sorry you went through that."

Reflection

- How do I respond to stories that make me uncomfortable?
- Have I ever unintentionally questioned someone's experience?
- What would support without judgment look like in my specialty?

Affirmation: "I don't have to have all the answers. I just need to offer safety, empathy, and belief."

A Provider's Prayer

God, let me be a quiet refuge.
When words fail, let my presence speak.
When fear rises, let peace enter with me.
Help me respond with courage, calm, and care.
Let every patient feel believed, not broken.
Amen.

Chapter Five

Empower Recovery (E)

Because survivors don't need us to take over; they need us to give options.

When someone has experienced sexual violence, they've already had something stolen from them: Choice. Power. Control. Voice.

As healthcare providers, we don't restore that by making decisions *for* them. We restore it by making decisions *with* them.

The final pillar of R.I.S.E.—**Empower Recovery** reminds us that every encounter is an opportunity to return autonomy to the survivor. It starts with information, is reinforced through options, and solidified through ongoing support. That is education and advocacy.

Empowerment is not a feeling. It's a practice. And it begins with the way we communicate.

What Empowerment Sounds Like

Trauma-informed empowerment isn't about telling a survivor they're "strong." It's about showing them they still have choices. It sounds like:

- "Here are a few options. You get to choose what works best for you."
- "We can stop or slow down anytime; just let me know."
- "Would you prefer to insert the speculum yourself, or would you like me to do it?"
- "We can schedule a follow-up—or not. You decide what feels right."

- "You're in charge of this visit. I'm here to guide, not push."

Each of these phrases gives something back: **power.**

The Danger of Assumptions

Even well-meaning providers can unintentionally disempower patients by assuming what's best for them:

- "You *should* report this."
- "This exam is required."
- "If you don't do this now, you'll regret it."
- "Don't worry, it's no big deal."

Survivors often internalize these statements as: *"I'm not being heard."* or *"I don't really have a choice."*

The moment we assume, we risk repeating the loss of control they've already endured.

The Power of Plain Language

Educating survivors means offering clear, honest, jargon-free explanations; even when we're busy.

Before a procedure:

"I'm going to walk you through each step. You'll know exactly what's coming and why it matters."

If the patient seems hesitant:

"Would it help to pause and go over what this means again?"

Even a 2-minute explanation can mean the difference between re-traumatization and relief.

Scenario: A Clinic Visit With Options

Kendra, a 29-year-old woman, is at the clinic for a follow-up after an ER visit. The nurse practitioner, informed by the notes, gently explains:

"I know the ER visit might've been overwhelming. Today, we'll only do what feels safe. I'll explain each step, why they are recommended, and we can stop or skip anything you don't want to do. You're in the lead here."

Kendra nods, tearful. No one's ever said that to her before.

That's trauma-informed advocacy in action.

Advocacy Beyond the Room

Empowerment also means advocating within the system:

- Making sure referral options include trauma-trained providers
- Ensuring patients know they can say "no" at any point
- Speaking up when policies feel coercive or unsafe
- Asking administrators to adopt trauma-informed protocols
- Ensuring accessibility: Is the handout inclusive? Is the language respectful of gender, race, and ability?

When you advocate for trauma-informed practices, you're not just helping the patient in front of you. You're creating a **culture** that protects the next one, too.

Sample Empowerment Language (By Specialty)

Primary Care/Internal Medicine

- "Here's what I'm recommending and why. What are your thoughts?"
- "Do you want time to decide before we proceed?"

Dentistry

- "Would you like a signal to pause if anything becomes uncomfortable?"

- "Would music or another form of distraction help during this part?"

Pediatrics

- "You get to choose. Should we check your ears or heartbeat first?"
- "You can tell me to stop anytime."

OBGYN

- "You're in control of this entire exam. Want to walk through each step together?"
- "Would you prefer a nurse in the room, or some privacy?"

Action Steps

Provide Choices at Every Stage

Not just in procedures, but in **scheduling**, **support people**, **treatment options**, and pace.

Normalize Questions

Say: "It's okay to ask questions at any point. Nothing is off-limits."

Offer Resources Without Pressure

Instead of "You need to see a counselor," try:

"There are some amazing resources if you ever want them. Would you like me to share a few?"

Affirm Their Voice After a disclosure:

"You did something powerful by speaking up. That was your choice, and it shows strength and resilience."

Reflection

- Do I speak in a way that encourages choice or compliance?

- When was the last time I paused to ask a patient what they *need* from me, rather than what I need from them?
- Am I actively advocating for a system that honors survivors?

Affirmation: "I don't rescue. I empower. I don't direct. I walk beside."

A Provider's Prayer

God,

Let me never forget that this body in front of me holds a story I may never know.

Teach me to offer options, not orders.

Let my words restore dignity, not dictate.

May I remember that healing is not mine to give, but it is mine to protect.

Amen.

Chapter Six

What Trauma-Informed Protocols Look Like

Because safety shouldn't depend on who's working that day.

Trauma-informed care is not just a mindset; it must be a method. While personal empathy can transform a moment, it's consistent, systemic practice that transforms outcomes.

That's where protocols come in.

Without clearly defined, trauma-informed protocols, care becomes unpredictable. Survivors are left hoping they'll get someone kind. Providers are left guessing. And small mistakes can lead to considerable harm.

Protocols ensure that *every patient,* no matter the day, provider, or setting, receives care that respects their dignity, autonomy, and safety.

Why Protocols Matter for Survivors

Survivors thrive on predictability. They need to know:

- What's going to happen
- Who's going to be present
- What options they have

- That they can stop at any time
- That they won't be judged if they say no
- What's going to happen next

Protocols make this consistent.

When your team has trauma-informed processes in place—from check-in to follow-up—you're not just protecting the patient. You're protecting your staff from burnout, confusion, and liability. Additionally, you're potentially improving your overall satisfaction scores.

A Trauma-Informed Protocol Is...

- Clear
- Written
- Staff-wide
- Inclusive of all roles (from security to admin to clinicians)
- Reviewed regularly
- Survivor-centered
- Grounded in informed choice, not just compliance

It is *not* just a poster in the breakroom or a one-time training.

Sample Trauma-Informed Protocol Elements

Here are sample protocols you can adapt for any clinic, hospital, private practice, or community health center.

1. Intake & Registration Protocol:

- Avoid asking invasive or trauma-related questions unless clinically necessary.

- An algorithm for staff to follow when a survivor enters your setting
- Do not require survivors to re-explain their story multiple times.
- Ask: "Would you prefer to complete your intake in writing, online, or verbally?"
- Train front desk staff to maintain respectful tone, avoid rushing, and honor the patients choices.

2. Room Preparation Protocol:

- Prepare all materials before the patient enters.
- Offer a clean gown with full coverage.
- Provide privacy to undress.
- Place a soft, folded blanket on the table if possible.
- Allow the patient to choose seating or lying position when appropriate.
- Ensure the door or curtain can close completely, if the survivor chooses.

3. Consent & Communication Protocol:

- Consent is ongoing, not one-time.
- Before touching the patient, always ask: "Is it okay if I...?" or "Would you like me to explain this part first?"
- Let the patient know they can pause or stop the exam at any point.
- Use clear, respectful language.

4. Response to Disclosure Protocol:

- Listen without judgment or interruption.
- Respond with validation: "Thank you for telling me. That took courage."

- Offer support: "Would you like to know what resources are available?"
- Do not pressure reporting.
- Document using the patient's language, not assumptions or summaries.
- Follow state-specific guidelines for mandated reporting and referrals. Know the laws in your state.

5. Follow-Up and Continuity Protocol:

- Offer the option of a same-gender provider if the survivor prefers and is available.
- Allow the patient to schedule with the same clinician if they choose.
- Provide written information on referrals (SANE programs, community crisis centers, therapy, advocacy centers, health department).
- Offer to connect them to a trauma-informed provider or resource in real-time.
- Include trauma-informed care notes in EMR (with consent), e.g., "prefers gentle communication," "anxious during exams," "requested nurse or suport person in room."

Institutional Culture: Beyond the Exam Room

Trauma-informed protocols also shape **team culture**.

- **Security staff** should be trained to de-escalate without intimidation.
- **Housekeeping teams** should know the importance of maintaining visual privacy.
- **Billing staff** should avoid harsh collection practices or language like "noncompliant."
- **Leadership** should model trauma-informed communication in staff meetings,

emails, and policy decisions.

When trauma-informed care becomes a shared standard, patients feel safer, staff provide care with confidence and compassion, feel supported, resulting in decreased staff burnout and turnover.

Scenario: The Clinic With a Protocol

At Harmony Family Practice, trauma-informed care is more than a buzzword. They've implemented protocols across every department:

- Front desk staff ask, "Do you have any accessibility or comfort preferences today?"
- All clinicians verbalize each step and ask for consent before beginning.
- Rooms have privacy signage and calming artwork.
- Each patient receives a handout titled: "You Are In Control of Your Care."

One patient, a survivor of childhood abuse, writes in a follow-up survey:
"I never thought I could feel safe in a medical setting again. But here, I felt seen, not just examined."

Action Steps

Audit your current patient flow. Where are the potential triggers? Where is consent assumed instead of given?

Draft or revise protocols using survivor input and staff feedback.

Train everyone, not just medical staff. Trauma-informed care is an all-team effort—from first contact to discharge and beyond.

Reinforce protocols regularly during huddles, onboarding, and evaluations.

Adapt for different specialties. What works for dentistry may differ from OB/GYN—but the principles stay the same.

Reflection

- Does our practice rely on individual providers to "get it right," or do we have systems that support safety?
- Do our protocols honor patient autonomy, or just protect liability?
- Where can we improve consistency in our trauma-informed practices?

Affirmation: "Safety shouldn't be a gamble. My care is consistent, compassionate, and prepared."

A Provider's Prayer

God,

May our site be a refuge.
Not just a place for treatment,
but a place where healing begins.
Let our protocols reflect Your love—steady, respectful, and full of grace.
May every system we create protect the dignity of those we serve.
Amen.

Chapter Seven

Specialty Spotlights

Trauma-informed care is not one-size-fits-all, but it is every provider's responsibility.

Sexual assault does not discriminate. It impacts children, adults, men, women, LGBTQ+ individuals, and people across every race, culture, and socioeconomic status. Survivors show up *everywhere.* In clinics, hospitals, dental offices, mobile units, therapy sessions, and school health centers.

That means *every specialty* is a frontline for trauma-informed care.

This chapter explores how the R.I.S.E. framework and the 4 R's of trauma-informed care apply in diverse healthcare settings—offering practical tools, language swaps, and real-world examples for each.

Because wherever there are patients, there are survivors. And they deserve to feel safe.

Dentistry & Oral Surgery

Why It Matters

The mouth is one of the most **common sites of trauma** in sexual violence, especially for male survivors and children. Dental exams can echo past abuse, both physically and psychologically.

Common Triggers

- Phrases like "open wide" or "this won't hurt"
- Lying flat with someone standing over them

- Hands near the mouth
- Gag reflexes triggering flashbacks

Trauma-Informed Practices

- Let patients signal when to pause (e.g., raising a hand)
- Offer a mirror so they can see what's happening
- Narrate every step with calm, respectful language
- Avoid using humor to downplay discomfort
- Allow them to sit up periodically
- Respect refusal without pressure

Suggested phrase: "I'll talk you through what I'm doing, but you're in control. We can stop anytime."

Pediatrics & Adolescent Care

Why It Matters

Children may not have the language to disclose abuse, but their behavior tells a story. Pediatric providers are uniquely positioned to detect trauma early, but they must be trained to recognize and respond with care.

Common Signs

- Avoidance of touch
- Overly compliant or overly aggressive behavior
- Regression, toileting issues, somatic complaints
- Fear of undressing or being alone with a provider

Trauma-Informed Practices

- Ask the child's permission when appropriate
- Offer choices: "Should we check your ears or throat first?"
- Never force physical exams—especially genital exams
- Let them stay partially clothed if possible
- Collaborate with caregivers but prioritize the child's emotional safety
- Use language they understand without minimizing their fear

Suggested phrase: "You're the boss of your body. If something feels scary, we'll take a break."

OBGYN & Reproductive Health

Why It Matters

This specialty sees some of the highest rates of patient re-traumatization. Pelvic exams, pregnancy care, and fertility treatment can all evoke memories of sexual assault.

Common Challenges

- High rates of noncompliance due to fear, not irresponsibility
- Patients not returning for follow-ups
- Avoidance of birth control or STI testing due to shame

Trauma-Informed Practices

- Offer self-insertion of instruments when possible
- Allow patient to wear socks or a drape for dignity

- Verbalize each step and check in frequently
- Offer same-gender providers when requested
- Use body-positive, shame-free language
- Avoid rushed exams or dismissive comments

Suggested phrase: "Would you like me to explain what's next, or would you prefer we take it slow and check in as we go?"

Internal Medicine & Family Practice

Why It Matters

This is often where survivors first interact with healthcare post-assault—**years later**, if at all. Many survivors present with chronic health issues rooted in unresolved trauma.

Common Presentations

- Chronic pain, fatigue, or GI symptoms with no clear origin
- Substance use, insomnia, anxiety
- Distrust of the system or frequent provider switching
- Over-apologizing or excessive defensiveness

Trauma-Informed Practices

- Screen for trauma history gently: "Has anything ever happened that makes exams uncomfortable?"
- Normalize mental health referrals without shame
- Use open-ended questions and offer autonomy over the agenda
- Avoid "tough love" language like "You just need to..."

Suggested phrase: "You're the expert on your body. I'm here to partner with you."

Emergency Medicine & Urgent Care

Why It Matters

Survivors often come to the ER after an assault, or for unrelated reasons, only to encounter triggers. Emergency providers are key gatekeepers of safety, validation, and referral.

Common Challenges

- High-pressure environment sometimes makes empathy challenging
- Risk of retraumatization with invasive procedures or hurried questioning
- Patients may be in shock or unable to speak

Trauma-Informed Practices

- Slow down when possible, even if briefly
- Avoid forcing decisions. Offer choices, not demands
- If assault is disclosed, call for a SANE nurse if one is on site, or an advocate immediately. Ensure you have a protocol for staff to follow when disclosures are made.
- If no SANE is available, document clearly and never minimize the report.
- Follow next steps if you have a protocol. If you don't have a protocol, it's time to change that.
- Be mindful of tone and body language

Suggested phrase: "You've been through something hard. You get to decide what happens next. I'm here to help."

Mental & Behavioral Health

Why It Matters

While this is the space where trauma is often unpacked, even mental health providers can unintentionally retraumatize through language, silence, or power dynamics.

Common Missteps

- Pushing for disclosure too early
- Pathologizing survivor responses
- Assuming verbal fluency equals emotional readiness

Trauma-Informed Practices

- Let the patient guide the pace
- Focus on regulation and trust before content
- Avoid language that implies "brokenness"
- Remind patients that trauma is a *response,* not a weakness

Suggested phrase: "We'll go at your pace. You get to decide what healing looks like."

School-Based & Community Clinics

Why It Matters

These are often *first access points* for young survivors. Staff may lack formal training but still have life-changing influence.

Common Needs

- Confidential space
- Mandated reporting awareness

- Cultural humility and nonjudgmental support

Trauma-Informed Practices

- Use calm tone and neutral language
- Acknowledge feelings without pushing for details
- Clearly explain confidentiality limits before beginning
- Connect with trusted community-based resources

Suggested phrase: "You're not in trouble. Thank you for sharing. Would you like to talk about what happens next?"

Private Practice & Concierge Medicine

Why It Matters

Even in high-end or boutique settings, survivors walk through the door. Trauma doesn't discriminate based on income or appearance.

Trauma-Informed Practices

- Include trauma-informed messaging on your website and forms
- Create soft, non-clinical environments where possible
- Offer personalized safety plans and continuity with providers
- Avoid invalidating concerns based on perceived stability or success

Suggested phrase: "We're here to support your whole self; including the parts of your story you haven't told yet."

Final Thoughts

Trauma-informed care is not about being perfect. It's about being present. Every specialty has a role to play. Every provider has the ability to reduce harm and increase hope.

When survivors know they are **safe**, **believed**, and **respected**, healing becomes possible, even in the most clinical of spaces.

Reflection

- What specialty-specific practices can I adjust to better support survivors?
- Are there phrases I regularly use that might be unknowingly harmful?
- How can I bring trauma-informed awareness into my team or specialty?

Affirmation: "I don't just treat symptoms. I create safety. My specialty is a sanctuary."

A Provider's Prayer

God,

Let my specialty be more than a skillset,
let it be a shelter.
May I see the sacred in every patient,
and treat every visit as a chance to restore dignity.
Where trauma has spoken loudly,
let my presence speak peace and healing.
Amen.

Chapter Eight

When a Patient Discloses

You may be the first safe person they've ever told.

Most survivors never report. Many never tell anyone. And for those who do disclose, healthcare providers are often the first people to hear it.

How we respond in those moments matters deeply. A survivor who is brave enough to share, even part of their story, is watching for your reaction:

- Do you believe me?
- Will you judge me?
- Am I safe now?

A trauma-informed response is not complicated, but it must be intentional. In this chapter, we'll walk through how to recognize, receive, document, and refer after a disclosure—verbally or otherwise.

Because no matter your role, if you work with patients, you need to be ready.

What Disclosure May Look Like

Disclosures can be:

- **Direct:** "I was raped." or "I was sexually assaulted."
- **Indirect:** "Something happened when I was a kid." or "I don't like being

touched." or "I had a bad experience once."

- Non-verbal: Crying during an exam, freezing, dissociating, flinching, becoming agitated or withdrawn without clear cause

If it feels like a disclosure, respond like it is. You don't need proof to offer compassion.

The First Moments Matter Most

A survivor has just made themselves vulnerable. Your job is ***not*** to investigate, interrogate, or even ask for details. Your job is to:

- Stay calm
- Stay grounded
- Respond with empathy
- Preserve their control

What to Say

- "Thank you for trusting me with that."
- "I believe you."
- "That shouldn't have happened to you."
- "You're not alone."
- "You're in control of what happens next."
- "Would it be okay if I shared some support options?"

What NOT to Say

- "Are you sure?"

- "Why didn't you tell anyone sooner?"
- "That sounds confusing."
- "What were you wearing?"
- "Do you want to report it?" (as a first question)
- "We still need to finish the exam."

Grounding Yourself in the Moment

Disclosures can be emotionally intense for the provider too. You may feel sad, shocked, helpless, or angry. That's normal.

Breathe. Plant your feet. Stay present. Stay regulated.

If needed, say, "Thank you for sharing that with me. I'm just taking a moment to make sure I respond in a helpful way."

You don't have to get it perfect. You just have to be real.

Scenario: A Routine Visit, a Life-Altering Moment

Dr. Han, a pediatrician, notices her thirteen-year-old patient becoming unusually quiet and tearful during a scoliosis screening. She gently asks, "Are you okay? Would you like to pause?"

The child hesitates, then whispers, "I hate when people touch me."

Dr. Han doesn't push. She kneels beside her and says, "Thank you for telling me that. I want you to feel safe here. We can take a break and talk about it, if you want to."

Mom was quiet, but accepts the referral the doctor later provides. During the follow up visit, the child discloses more to the therapist. That moment opened the door to healing and justice.

When You're a Mandated Reporter

Note: Laws vary from state to state.

In many settings, providers are required to report abuse of:

- Minors
- Vulnerable adults
- Elderly individuals
- Patients in institutional care

Disclosing your role as a mandated reporter should happen *BEFORE* a disclosure if possible.

"I want you to know, if you ever share something that makes me concerned for your safety or someone else's, I may need to get help. But I'll walk through it with you."

If you *do* need to report, stay calm. Involve the patient, when appropriate. Explain what will happen, and reassure them they're not in trouble.

Documentation Do's and Don'ts

What you write matters—for legal, clinical, and ethical reasons.

Do:

- Use the patient's exact words in quotes
- Document only what was said or observed, not your interpretation
- Record time, date, and your response
- Note referrals or follow-up actions

Don't:

- Use clinical shorthand that minimizes (e.g., "appears hysterical")
- Diagnose trauma without confirmation
- Insert personal opinions or judgments

Example: Patient stated, "I was sexually assaulted last year."

I responded, "Thank you for telling me. I believe you."

Offered list of local support services. Patient declined further assistance today. Will follow up at next visit.

Referring With Care

Disclosure is not the end. It's the beginning of what can be a long healing process. Your referral might be the bridge to that healing.

Best Practices:

- Offer at least two trauma-informed resources (e.g., community crisis center, Health Department, therapist, advocacy center)
- Provide written and verbal options
- Never pressure a patient to report to law enforcement
- Let them decide when/if to engage follow-up services
- Offer to help them make the call, if they want support

Action Steps

Prepare before it happens: Train staff to respond consistently to disclosures. Keep referral resources updated and accessible.

Practice grounding techniques: Know how to regulate yourself in emotionally intense situations.

Use compassionate scripts: Memorize a few key phrases so you're ready.

Treat disclosures as sacred: Even if you're busy. Even if it's inconvenient. These moments matter.

Reflection

- If a patient were to disclose to me tomorrow, how would I respond?

- Do I feel confident in what to say and do next?
- Does my documentation reflect empathy as well as accuracy?

Affirmation: "I don't need to have all the answers. I just need to hold space with care."

Provider's Prayer

God,

If a patient opens their pain to me,
let my words bring calm, not confusion.
Let my hands bring steadiness, not fear.
Let my presence be proof that trust is still possible.
Teach me to listen more than I speak
and to respond with truth, tenderness, and strength.
Amen.

Chapter Nine

Vicarious Trauma, Burnout, And Boundaries

You can't pour from an empty cup—and you shouldn't be expected to.

Trauma-informed care requires deep presence, steady patience, and a soft place for someone else's pain to land.

But what happens when that pain begins to take up space inside *you*?

When you bear witness to trauma day after day; especially without enough support, something happens. You begin to feel tired in a way that rest doesn't fix. Numb to stories that once moved you. Resentful of the work that once gave you purpose.

This is more than stress. This is **vicarious trauma**. And if left unchecked, it can become burnout.

In this chapter, we'll talk about how to recognize the signs in yourself, how to stay emotionally regulated, and how to protect your peace without abandoning your calling.

Because you deserve care too.

What Is Vicarious Trauma?

Vicarious trauma is the internal shift that happens when providers absorb the emotional weight of their patients' trauma. It's not weakness. It's a *normal occupational hazard* for caregivers, especially those working closely with survivors of sexual violence.

You didn't experience the trauma yourself, but part of your nervous system begins to act like you did.

Some Signs of Vicarious Trauma

- Difficulty sleeping or relaxing after emotionally intense encounters
- Feeling detached, cynical, or numb toward patients
- Loss of empathy or compassion fatigue
- Intrusive thoughts about a patient's experience
- Avoidance of work or certain procedures
- Physical symptoms (headaches, stomachaches, fatigue)
- Emotional exhaustion, dread, or questioning your role

If you've found yourself thinking, *"I just don't have anything left to give,"*—this chapter is for you.

Burnout Isn't Just About Workload

Burnout often gets blamed on long hours. But for providers who work with trauma, the *emotional weight* is the real burden.

Burnout can happen when:

- You're expected to give more than you're resourced to deliver
- You don't have space to process what you hear
- You're treated like a machine, not a human
- You have poor work-life balance
- You neglect Self-care

You can't trauma-inform your care if you're constantly *operating from survival mode.* You're driving on *E.*

Boundaries Are Not Selfish

You don't need to be available 24/7 to prove you care. You don't need to say yes to every patient, every extra shift, or every emotional request. You shouldn't be required to pour out more than you have, without space for yourself.

Boundaries don't push people away; they preserve your ability to show up with empathy.

Every time you say:

- "I need a moment to breathe,"
- "That's not something I can do right now,"
- "Let me refer you to someone who can help,"

you are modeling what healthy regulation and self-respect look like.

And survivors need to see that too.

Regulation Starts With You

One of the most powerful tools you have in trauma-informed care isn't your clinical skill; it's your nervous system. When you stay calm, the patient feels safer. When you're grounded, you become a regulated presence in their dysregulated world.

Daily Regulation Tools

- Take three grounding breaths between patients
- Do a full-body scan when you feel tension
- Use a transition ritual between work and home (e.g., music, prayer, deep breathing in the car)

- Spend time with beauty: nature, art, stillness
- Unplug from trauma-related media after hours

Even two to three minutes of intentional regulation can shift your internal state.

Scenario: Compassion Without Collapse

Nurse Tara has worked in the ER for twelve years. She's known for her empathy, but lately, she finds herself going numb. A survivor tells her a heartbreaking story, and Tara nods, but feels nothing.

At home, she can't sleep. She cries at commercials and dreads going back to work. She begins to question whether she's in the right field.

Her supervisor notices and recommends a peer support group. Tara hesitates, but eventually joins. She hears another nurse say, "You don't have to carry it alone."

That's the beginning of her return.

Organizational Responsibility

While individual boundaries are vital, *burnout is not just a personal issue. It may be a system failure.*

Leaders must:

- Normalize conversations about secondary trauma
- Offer space for debriefing and emotional processing
- Provide access to therapy and peer support
- Protect breaks and reasonable workloads
- Avoid punishing staff for needing mental health days

If you're expected to absorb pain without support, you're being harmed too.

Action Steps

Acknowledge your limits. You are not a vessel with infinite capacity. Recognizing your threshold is wise, not weak.

Develop a self-regulation plan. What practices help you reset between difficult encounters? How do you refill your own cup?

Use your voice. Advocate for policies that protect both patients and staff.

Build community. Trauma is heavy and you shouldn't try to carry it alone. Join a peer group or mentorship circle.

Seek professional support if needed. Therapy isn't just for patients. Providers need safe spaces too. Access your employer's wellness resources and employee assistance programs (EAP).

Reflection

- How am I *really* doing—emotionally, mentally, spiritually, and physically?
- Do I feel like I have to carry everything myself?
- Where in my life could I create more space to rest and recover?

Affirmation: "I serve with heart, but I am not the healing. I am a helper, not a savior. My limits deserve compassion too."

A Provider's Prayer

God,

I want to serve with joy again.
I want to feel again—without breaking.
Help me lay down what isn't mine to carry.
Help me rest when I need rest,
breathe when I need breath,
and know that even when I pause,
the world will keep turning.
Let me be faithful in my calling
without forgetting my own humanity.
Amen.

Chapter Ten

Your Role in the Healing Journey

You don't need to fix the past; you just need to show up differently now.

You may never hear the full story. You may never know what happened behind closed doors, or how deeply the trauma runs. But you still have the power to shape a survivor's future; with one moment of dignity, one trauma-informed choice, one safe interaction.

That's the quiet power of your role in the healing journey.

Whether you're a doctor, nurse, therapist, dentist, technician, assistant, or administrator your presence matters. You are not "just" a provider. You are part of someone's path to reclaiming their voice, their worth, and their peace.

You are an integral part of their restoration.

Healing Happens in Small Moments

We tend to think of healing as a long, dramatic process. But for many survivors, it starts in the simplest places:

- A receptionist who greets them by name and with kindness
- A nurse who doesn't rush when asking sensitive questions
- A dentist who pauses and says, "You're in control."
- A provider who listens, without looking away

- A staff member who says, "You did nothing wrong."

These are the moments that survivors remember—long after the appointment ends.

You Might Be the First Safe Person

So many survivors have been disbelieved, dismissed, or violated in places where they were supposed to be protected.

If you respond with respect and compassion, you may be the first safe person they've ever encountered in healthcare. The first one who didn't flinch at their story. The first one who didn't hurry them along. The first one who let them breathe.

And that changes everything.

The Ripple Effect of Trauma-Informed Care

When you respond with safety, empathy, and choice, you:

- Interrupt cycles of shame
- Prevent re-traumatization
- Increase patient retention and trust
- Support your colleagues by modeling good practice
- Create a culture that invites healing, not harm

And most importantly, you remind survivors of something they may have forgotten: **They are more than what happened to them. They are still worthy of gentle care.**

You're Not Alone in This Work

You don't have to carry the full weight of someone's healing. You are one part of a bigger story. A chapter. A turning point.

When you offer trauma-informed care, you plant a seed; one that may grow long after the patient leaves your setting.

"The doctor didn't change my life. But they showed me it was worth saving." —Survivor

Scenario: A New Narrative

Jasmine, a twenty-four-year-old survivor, avoided doctors for years after her assault. Her body didn't feel like hers, and every appointment felt invasive; like she was being assaulted all over again.

But this time was different.

The doctor asked for consent multiple times and gave her options. Spoke softly. Checked in. Paused when Jasmine froze. Offered support resources without pressure.

Jasmine left feeling something she hadn't felt in years: **hope**.

Action Steps

Stay curious. Keep learning about trauma, resilience, and survivor-centered care.

Mentor others. Share what you've learned with colleagues. Model what trauma-informed care looks like.

Revisit your "why." Why did you choose this work? Let that mission ground you when things feel heavy.

Celebrate your impact. Healing is not always visible; but it's real.

Reflection

- Who taught me how to be a safe presence?
- How do I want my patients to feel when they leave my care?
- What legacy of safety, dignity, and compassion do I want to leave in this profession?

Affirmation: "I am a witness to resilience. A protector of dignity. A partner in healing. That is enough."

A Final Prayer for Providers

God,

Thank You for the sacred trust of this work.
Let me never forget the weight and wonder
of holding another person's story.
When I feel tired, remind me that presence is power.
When I feel small, remind me that healing happens in moments.
And when I forget why I started,
bring me back to love.
Let every patient feel seen.
Let every word reflect compassion.
Let my care be a seed—planted in hope, watered with grace.
Amen.

Chapter Eleven

A Call to RISE

This is more than a book. It's your invitation to begin.

As you have read throughout the book, trauma isn't rare. It's not isolated to a certain age group, gender, socioeconomic status, sexual orientation, or zip code. It's in your waiting room. On your exam table. In your dental chair. In your hands.

Assume ***EVERY*** patient is a survivor.

Every day, survivors show up in your settings hoping this time will be different—this time, they'll be seen, not sized up. Heard, not hurried. Treated, not triggered.

And now, thanks to you, that hope is not misplaced.

You've read this book because you care. You want to do better, be better, and lead with compassion. That alone sets you apart.

But don't stop here.

Let your learning become leadership. Let your awareness become action. Let your clinical skill be matched by your trauma-informed survivor-centered heart.

You can't go back and change someone's past. But you *can* change what happens next. You can change the narrative. The tone. The outcome.

And in doing so, you become more than a provider. You become a partner in someone's healing.

So keep rising. Keep advocating. Keep creating the kind of care every patient deserves.

Trauma-informed care isn't a "special add-on." It's the foundation for ethical, respectful healthcare that benefits every patient, every member of staff, not just survivors.

Trauma-informed care is about anticipating needs, not just reacting to distress.

The work begins with one moment. One room. One choice. Rise with us.

Glossary of Key Terms

4R's of Trauma-Informed Care

The four foundational principles (Realize, Recognize, Respond, Resist) established by SAMHSA form the base of trauma-informed practice.

ACEs (Adverse Childhood Experiences

Potentially traumatic events that occur in childhood—such as abuse, neglect, or household dysfunction—that can have long-term effects on health and behavior.

Disclosure

When a patient voluntarily shares that they have experienced sexual assault or trauma. Disclosure may occur verbally or through non-verbal cues.

Empowerment

The process of restoring control and autonomy to survivors by involving them in their care decisions and honoring their boundaries.

Flat Affect

A limited or absent display of emotion often seen in trauma survivors. It may include minimal facial expressions or monotone speech. Providers should view this as a possible trauma response rather than indifference.

Informed Consent

Ensuring that patients are fully informed about their options, procedures, and potential risks before voluntarily agreeing to treatment.

Re-Traumatization

When interactions, procedures, or settings unintentionally remind a survivor of their trauma, causing renewed distress.

R.I.S.E. Framework

A trauma-informed care model that empowers healthcare teams to provide survivor-centered care:

R – Recognize trauma, I – Initiate safe care, S – Support healing, E – Empower recovery

SAMHSA's Principles of Trauma-Informed Care

The six core principles: Safety; Trustworthiness & Transparency; Peer Support; Collaboration & Mutuality; Empowerment, Voice, & Choice; and Cultural, Historical, & Gender Awareness.

Survivor-Centered Care

An approach that prioritizes the survivor's safety, dignity, and autonomy in all healthcare interactions.

Trauma-Informed Care (TIC)

A framework that recognizes the prevalence and impact of trauma, integrating practices that promote safety, trust, and healing.

Triggers

Words, actions, smells, or sensations that cause a person to relive aspects of their trauma.

Vicarious Trauma

The emotional toll that healthcare providers experience after repeated exposure to patients' trauma, which can lead to compassion fatigue or burnout.

Appendix A

Trauma-Informed Provider Self-Assessment

Use this reflection tool to evaluate your trauma-informed readiness.

On a scale of 1 (rarely) to 5 (consistently), how often do I...

Statement	1 2 3 4 5
1. I ask for consent before every procedure—even routine ones	
2. I offer choices and honor patient preferences when possible	
3. I pause when patients show signs of distress, even if subtle	
4. I use language that is clear, respectful, and free from medical jargon	
5. I remain regulated and calm during difficult patient interactions	
6. I respond to disclosures without judgment or rushing to fix the situation.	
7. I avoid making assumptions about a patient's background or history	
8. I recognize the signs of burnout or vicarious trauma in myself	
9. My practice has clear protocols for trauma-informed care	
10. I regularly seek opportunities to grow in trauma-informed practice	

Appendix B

Sample Scripts for Trauma-Informed Language

When starting an exam:

"I'll explain each step before we begin. You're in control and can pause at any time."

When observing distress:

"I notice this feels uncomfortable. Want to take a moment or talk through what's next?"

When a patient discloses trauma:

"Thank you for trusting me. That shouldn't have happened to you. Would you like to know what support options are available?"

When offering options:

"There are a few ways we can approach this. Let's talk about what feels safest to you."

Appendix C

Suggested Trauma-Informed Room Checklist

- Room is clean, uncluttered, and softly lit
- Gown or covering offers full dignity
- Patient has privacy to undress
- Door closes fully and locks if needed
- Provider sits at eye level
- Materials are prepared beforehand
- Consent is requested for each step
- A trauma-informed poster or affirmation is visible
- Optional: calming music, warm blanket, or patient distraction tool

Appendix D

Resources And References

The following resources have been carefully curated to support healthcare professionals and survivors alike. They include foundational trauma-informed care frameworks, practical implementation tools, and survivor-centered organizations. Because trauma knows no borders, this appendix features both U.S.-based and Jamaican resources—reflecting the global reach of trauma and the universal need for compassion, safety, and restoration in care. Whether you are a healthcare provider, educator, or survivor seeking guidance, these organizations and references offer pathways to understanding, healing, and empowerment.

Foundational Frameworks

SAMHSA. Trauma-Informed Care in Behavioral Health Services. Rockville, MD: Substance Abuse and Mental Health Services Administration, 2014.

Fallot, R. & Harris, M. Creating Cultures of Trauma-Informed Care (CCTIC): A Self-Assessment and Planning Protocol. Community Connections, Washington, D.C.

Healthcare Implementation Resources

Center for Health Care Strategies. Trauma-Informed Care Implementation Resource Center. Available at: https://www.traumainformedcare.chcs.org

National Child Traumatic Stress Network (NCTSN). Medical Traumatic Stress Toolkit for Health Care Providers.

U.S.-Based Survivor Support Resources

RAINN (Rape, Abuse & Incest National Network): 1-800-656-4673: Website: https://www.rainn.org

NSVRC (National Sexual Violence Resource Center): Website: https://www.nsvrc.org

CDC (Center for Disease Control and Prevention): Website: https://www.cdc.gov/

VSC (Victim Service Center of Central Florida): Website: https://www.victimservicecenter.org

ACEs Matter: Website: https://www.acesmatter.org

SVI (Samaritan Village): Website: https://www.samaritanvillage.net

Jamaican Resources

Woman Inc. Crisis Centre Hotline – 24/7 hotline for survivors of sexual violence, interpersonal violence, and trafficking. Counseling and limited shelter available. Hotline: 876-929-2997: Website: https://findahelpline.com/organizations/woman-inc-crisis-centre-hotline

Circle of Care Jamaica – Holistic psychosocial and empowerment services for survivors of abuse: Website: https://circleofcarejamaica.org

She Speaks (Angelic Ladies Society) – Advocacy, awareness, and survivor support programs for women and girls: Website: https://angelicladiessociety.org/shespeaks

CPFSA (Child Protection & Family Services Agency) – National agency for child welfare, with trauma-informed psychotherapy programs for children. Website: https://www.childprotection.gov.jm

JFJ (Jamaicans for Justice) – Human rights organization offering legal advocacy and support for victims of abuse: Website: https://jamaicansforjustice.org/

J-FLAG (Jamaica Forum for Lesbians, All-Sexuals & Gays) – Provides legal support, advocacy, and safe spaces for LGBTQ+ individuals, including survivors of sexual violence. Website: https://www.jflag.org

Appendix E

Recommended Reading and Training

READING

- *The Body Keeps the Score;* Bessel van der Kolk, M.D.
- *What Happened to You?* by Dr. Bruce Perry and Oprah Winfrey
- *Trauma Stewardship by* Laura van Dernoot Lipsky
- *Who Says You Can't Heal? Overcoming and Thriving After Sexual Assault by* Marie McKenzie

TRAINING

- International Sexual Assault Coaching Institute (ISACI)
- Florida Council Against Sexual Violence (FCASV)
- Victim Service Center of Central Florida (VSC)
- Aces Matter

About the Author

Once silenced by the aftermath of sexual assault, Marie McKenzie has devoted her life to breaking the silence surrounding the most under reported crime. She supports survivors and equips healthcare providers with tools to deliver compassionate, trauma-informed care. To further this cause, she founded the International Sexual Assault Coaching Institute, a platform for advocacy, education, and transformation in the fight against sexual violence.

With over two and a half decades of experience as a registered nurse, including her role as a sexual assault nurse examiner in the clinical and community settings, Marie blends her professional expertise with the tools and techniques that facilitated her own healing journey.

Renowned for her award-winning and bestselling memoir, *Things That Keep Me Up At Night*, Marie chronicles her personal odyssey from sexual assault at the age of eleven to her triumphant transformation. Her book serves as a beacon of hope, encouraging others to find their voices, share their stories, seek support, and embrace a life imbued with purpose.

Marie doesn't shy away from her calling, proudly declaring, "My mission is to remove sexual assault from being the most under reported crime."

She previously served on the board of The Inner Truth Project, a nonprofit aiding survivors of sexual violence to reclaim their voices and heal. Former secretary of the Central Florida Writers & Publishers Guild, current board member for The Esther Alliance (formerly KISS, Inc), and the Florida Council Against Sexual Violence.

When Marie is not educating healthcare providers to care for survivors, she collaborates with various organizations dedicated to helping those affected by diverse traumas. She enjoys the vibrant life of Orlando, Florida, alongside her husband, George.

To contact the author: marielmckenzie@gmail.com

Linktree: https://linktr.ee/mckenziemariel

Other Books by the Author

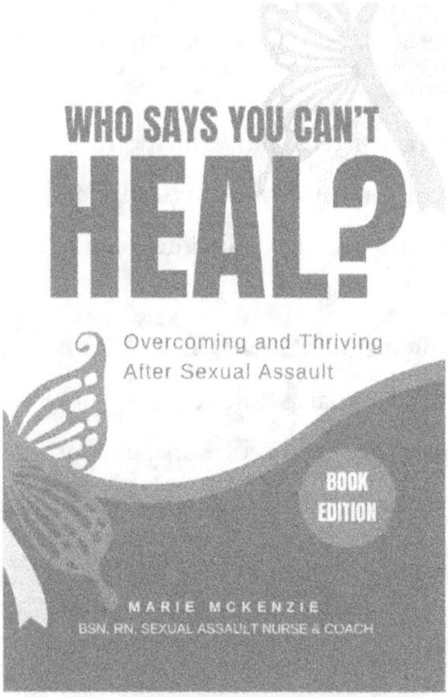

Who Says You Can't Heal? Overcoming and Thriving After Sexual Assault.

"Who Says You Can't Heal?" explores the profound process of developing the passion to heal and thrive after the harrowing experience of sexual assault. It aims to empower survivors and inspire resilience.

Inside these pages, you'll gain understanding, be reminded of self-love and self-compassion, find practical advice, process your pain, confront challenges, and emerge stronger than ever.

Whether you're navigating the complex emotions of guilt and shame, redefining intimacy, or learning to celebrate small victories, this book will guide you every step of the way.

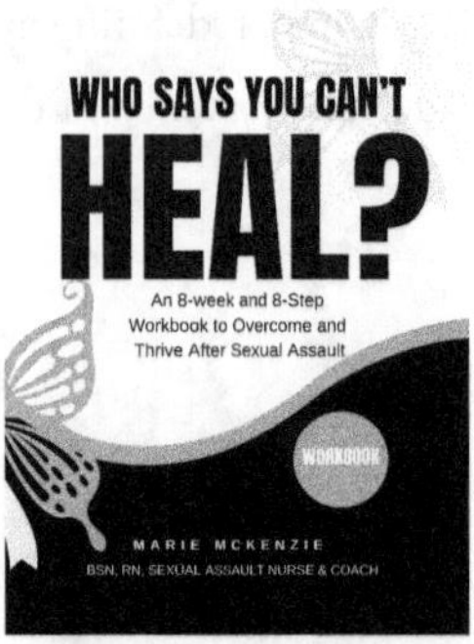

Who Says You Can't Heal? An 8-week and 8-Step Workbook to Overcome and Thrive After Sexual Assault

This workbook explores the profound process of developing the passion to heal and thrive after the harrowing experience of sexual assault. It aims to empower survivors and inspire resilience.

Inside these pages, you'll gain understanding, be reminded of self-love and self-compassion, process your pain, confront challenges, and emerge stronger than ever.

Whether you're navigating the complex emotions of guilt and shame, redefining intimacy, or learning to celebrate small victories, this workbook will guide you every step of the way.

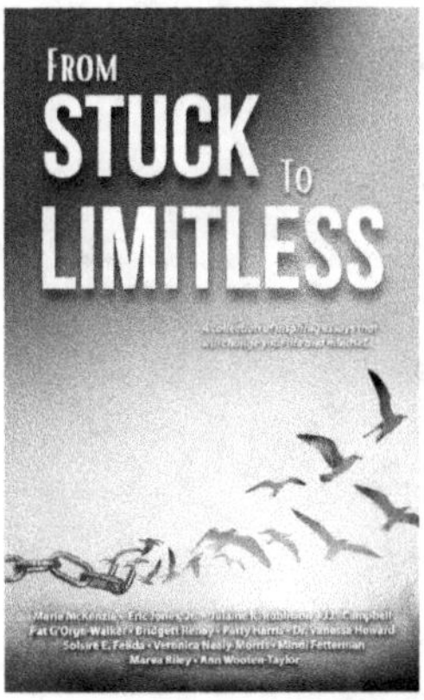

From Stuck to Limitless

Do you still harbor hurt and pain from past experiences?

From Stuck to Limitless is an anthology featuring individuals who share their harsh truths about trauma and survival—from childhood sexual and mental abuse, adult traumas, and debilitating health issues.

Through such truth-telling, we learn we are not alone and that it is only by sharing that we can heal ourselves and give hope to others.

So, get ready to pick up your copy of this impactful collection of essays from some of today's changemakers.

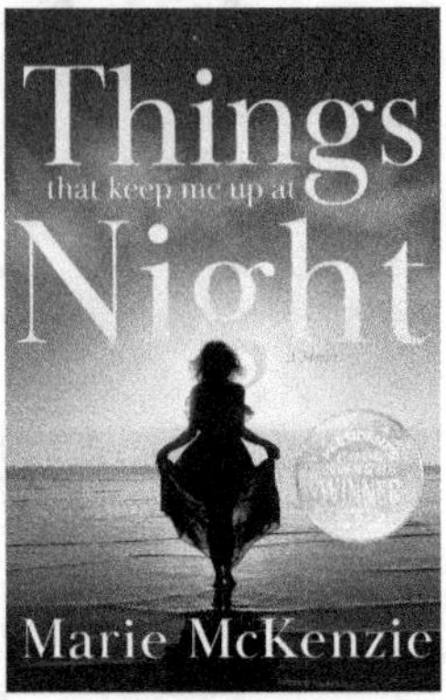

Things That Keep Me Up At Night

If you've ever wondered whether faith and determination are a recipe for success, *Things That Keep Me Up at Night* answers that question.

In this compelling memoir, McKenzie takes you on her journey from adversity to triumph.

From sexual assault at the age of eleven, she charts her path through the hills and valleys on the way to becoming a successful Registered Nurse. She pays tribute to the people who inspired, encouraged, and supported her through various stages of her life and career.

Her work as an advocate for victims of sexual assault and rape, domestic violence, and homelessness will encourage those who have been through similar experiences and need their hope restored.

www.ingramcontent.com/pod-product-compliance
Lightning Source LLC
LaVergne TN
LVHW022307200926
848481LV00004B/1240
9798988448273